SLEEP MATTERS

Improve Your Sleep, Improve Your Life

JENNIFER SPARKS

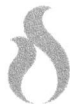

DISCLAIMER

As I am not a doctor, if you are suffering from sleep issues, I urge you to reach out to your doctor for additional supports. This book is not meant to replace medical advice. In cases of medical conditions that may be causing sleep issues, you will need help from a qualified professional.

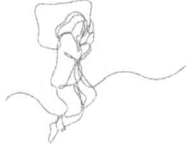

Introduction

I was a decent sleeper as a child. Although, when I was experiencing stress about anything significant my sleep became disruptive and I often would panic that I had not gotten any sleep and worry about how would I ever function without a solid night's sleep the next day. Once I moved into adulthood, I realized I could perform the day following a night of poor sleep, but I also learned that it took days to recover from that and I wasn't really on top of my game.

Then, my daughter became ill. At 12, she started having seizures, and our lives turned upside down. The impact of her illness and severity of seizure activity had a profound influence on my ability to fall asleep, stay asleep, and the quality of the sleep I had when I managed to finally drift off. I only needed to wake once to the sounds of her choking to believe that it was dangerous for me to sleep as her life was in danger.

My mental health began to suffer, and I became another person in terms of how I functioned, made decisions, and what I was able to tolerate before I entered a state of overwhelm. Before her illness and my newly acquired sleep dysfunction, I was a high functioning "get it done" type of person. I often was heavily committed to things and could move through heavy tasks loads without dropping any balls or being late with deliverables and obligations. I was incredibly focused and productive. And rested.

But everything changed. Not to mention the impact lack of sleep had on my hormones, eating habits, and my ability to take care of other elements in my life. I am still a recovering "dysfunctional sleeper" and work diligently to practice good sleep habits consistently because I realize it is a CRITICAL foundational piece to my overall wellbeing.

In this short read, I am going to share with you the things I have learned on my journey to healthier sleep and how I have integrated them into my life and home environment. Take from this collection of tips anything that resonates with you and leave what doesn't. If anything, I have learned there is never a one size fits all fix that works for everyone. Our lives, families, schedules, careers, environments and other activities all impact what and how these ideas may be integrated into daily sleep plans.

In the back of this booklet, I have also listed some additional resources that cover the topics of sleep, fatigue, and anti-sleep culture. If you are looking for more information, start there!

ONE

What Are We Told About Sleep?

Sleep has a bad rap. If we sleep too much, we are called lazy. But what is too much sleep? Sleep is a powerful natural state that allows our bodies and minds to rest, recover, and repair. Without good quality sleep, we are taking away a powerful foundation for health and wellness. When we do that, many parts of our lives can begin to suffer. But culturally, we do not value sleep, and it shows. How many times have you heard someone bragging about how little sleep they need to function at their peak? Or, how many times has the lack of sleep been overlooked as an issue?

What are your thoughts on sleep?

We may have been misled into thinking that if we sleep less, we can do more. ***What is true is that while we may do more, we do it more poorly than if we had been rested.*** If you subtract ninety minutes of sleep from your night, you will have reduced your cognitive function by a whopping thirty percent. No thanks.

And we are compromising our health and wellness to do this. Poor sleep has a direct impact on mind, body, moods, cognitive function, and our relationships with others. It impacts every aspect of our lives, and you do everything better with sleep.

Ideally, we would be striving for 7-8 hours of high quality, restorative sleep per night. Further, the best "performers" actually sleep more! They average 8.5 hours of sleep when the rest of the population is averaging 6.5 hours a night. Sleep correlates directly to success in all aspects of your life, yet is often overlooked as a wellness, management, and growth tool.

Sleep is powerful medicine. You can go four days without water, twenty-five days without food, and six days without sleep. It is a basic human need.

TWO

How Can We Optimize Sleep?

We need to openly discuss and value how important sleep is to our health. We need to accept that less sleep doesn't equate to more time to do things well. We need to understand the severe consequences of sleep deprivation. If you can change your sleep, you really can change your life and all aspects of it.

We need to prioritize sleep because sleep allows us to heal, rest, and reboot.

There is a stigma attached to sleeping, and we are taught that people who sleep are not successful or driven. **But, people who sleep are the smart ones, and they benefit from their choice to prioritize sleep.** They are more resilient, emotionally and mentally healthier, and they aren't cashing in their lifespan for less sleep. Have you have heard the saying, "You can sleep when you are dead?" Technically, you may be arriving there much more quickly if you do not allow yourself adequate sleep now.

How can we create a lifestyle that supports our need for quality sleep?

It doesn't matter what you are trying to do in your life if your sleep is suffering even if you are getting the suggested hours per night of sleep. If you are missing out on high quality sleep, all other efforts to improve your life and happiness will be less than optimized.

If you suffer from poor sleep habits or poor sleep quality, it can impact your weight, your brain function in terms of memory, focus, decision-making processes, your stress levels, mood, relationships, productivity, energy, and overall health. That's a significant hit.

In my case, I was always a good sleeper. I fell asleep quickly, and I stayed asleep. When children came on the scene, I was still able to fall back to sleep when they woke me, albeit I got fewer hours per night. I was functional most of the time. And then my daughter developed a seizure disorder, and my sleep was disrupted by shots of adrenaline, trips to the ER, middle of the night first aid, anxiety, and hyper-vigilance. It didn't matter that I worked Monday – Friday 8-4pm, I was ON all the time. When I was asleep, I had one foot on the floor, and I was listening for any abnormal sounds, and when I heard them, I got a shot of adrenalin that would have to work its way out of my body in the following hours, even if there was no real emergency. I was not getting the deep sleep I needed. There was no time for my body to repair itself, and it showed in all areas of my life.

THREE

I Didn't Realize How Much Sleep Mattered to My Health

What happened to my health and sleeping habits following my daughter's diagnosis was likely predictable by doctors, but no one said anything to me, and I hadn't even considered it as my focus was on taking care of her. I wish I had some warning or been sent out the door with some tips for how to keeping good sleep hygiene.

I did the best to keep the lid on this pot of "rapidly boiling life" issues. I was a single parent and the sole caregiver for my daughter. I continued to work full-time while trying to manage everything at home. Often work seemed like an escape from the chaos at home, but it wasn't. It was just a less personalized crisis zone, so it felt less urgent to me because no one could die there. But I always had my focus on what was going on at home and at one point while I was at work, I kept an eye on my daughter through a remote video feed to my phone. However, if she ever walked out of the frame and didn't come back, it didn't take long for panic to set in. Yes, I hired people watch her but she did not appreciate that as she was old enough to babysit other people's children. It was an odd age to require 24/7 supervision and felt like a huge breach of her privacy and independence but I was stuck.

I would come home from work, having checked in on her multiple times a day. Sometimes, I left work when she wouldn't answer the phone or was out of video feed zone because my anxiety would hit the roof as I imagined that she was laying on the floor unconscious. I felt like I was running on pure adrenalin, and I likely was. Often I would come home and have to deal with helping her learn how to manage her emotions, anxiety, and depression but I was depleted and my patience thin. And, then there were the seizures, first aid, ER visits, and all the associated "stuff" that comes along with this diagnosis.

There was no quality sleep. There was no downtime. There was no structure or routine or winding down at the end of the day rituals because seizures don't play by these rules. The best plans often went awry.

Over the next six years, I became increasingly impacted by these broken sleep patterns. I never discussed it with anyone, and just assumed I needed to figure it out. I also refused to take any sleep aids because I had deep fear if I fell asleep, I wouldn't hear her seizing, and I would not be able to help keep her safe.

I became anxious. I became indecisive. I became moody, and then I just turned my moods off completely and became disconnected. I gained weight. I made poor food choices. I was chronically dehydrated and over consumed caffeine around the clock because I had other responsibilities that I needed to deal with each day. I stopped exercising because I had no energy. I was depleted.

My doctor gave me seven sleeping pills. I took half of one and felt worse, so I never touched them again. I knew I had to figure it out on my own and I started researching everything and for the first time, began to value my own sleep as a lifestyle and wellness component.

FOUR

There Comes a Point Where the Madness Must Stop

In my story, there came the point where the doctors were able to stabilize my daughter's seizures, and once we had some breathing space, the first thing I did was take myself back to the basics. Had she not stabilized, I would have had to seriously consider some element of respite because I was in trouble from such extensive sleep deprivation.

I had to clean up the sleep. Then, I would work on the other things because I knew that the lack of proper sleep was messing with my health in more ways than one.

I had created a mess.

Mentally, emotionally, and physically. I was anxious, depressed, and jumpy. I couldn't make decisions, and I felt cognitively stuck. I would have mood swings, and I avoided people. I had gained weight and developed bad habits as a coping mechanism to stay awake when I needed sleep. Because of my reliance on caffeine, even when I did sleep, it wasn't deep sleep. I leaned heavily on the nightly glass or two of wine to fall asleep, but I tossed and turned as it metabolized. I had pets waking me up when I did manage to fall asleep, and my daughter also had horrible sleeping habits because of her anti-seizure medications so I could often hear her moving at night.

- What do your sleep habits look like?
- How dysfunctional do your sleep habits feel to you?
- Are you willing to restructure your life to make sleep a priority?
- What can you do to encourage regular sleep patterns?

FIVE

Are You Sleep Deprived?

Sleep deprivation can lead to many issues. Some you will associate with poor sleep and others you may not. Let's take a look at a few of them.

- Irritability
- Cognitive impairment
- Memory lapses or loss
- Impaired judgment and decision-making
- Severe yawning
- Hallucinations
- Symptoms similar to ADHD
- Poor immune system
- Risk of diabetes
- Increased heart rate variability
- Risk of heart disease
- Decreased reaction time
- Tremors
- Aches
- Risk of obesity

- Reduced body temperature
- Moodiness
- Increased hunger
- Increased safety risks

When you think that many of the items on this list can be prevented, you have to ask yourself WHY we, as a culture, do not value and promote high quality sleep habits?

SIX

Benefits of Proper Sleep

If you were to button down the hatches and do what you could to improve your sleeping habits, what improvements might you expect to begin seeing in your day to day health and wellness? Let's take a look.

- Improved memory
- Reduced risk for depression and anxiety
- Improved physical performance
- Sharpened attention
- Reduced stress
- Increased ability to heal
- Increased alertness
- Enhanced cognitive function
- Reduced inflammation
- Corrected hormone production
- Increased immune protection
- Increased creativity
- Decreased hunger

- Decreased cravings for high sugar, high-fat foods
- Extended life span

That list looks pretty good, doesn't it? Not only will proper sleep habits lead to better sleep and better health but much of danger we put ourselves in can be decreased by being well rested and alert.

SEVEN

When to Sleep

One of the first things I learned upon visiting my naturopathic doctor was that any sleep I could get from about ten in the evening until about two in the morning was worth double the sleep I would get after that. Also, mid-afternoon was a great time to nap if I was able to. She called them the golden hours.

Knowing this, I adjusted my routine to go to bed by ten pm so that I could get in some of the best quality of sleep. While I was still trying to establish deeper sleeping habits, I did continue to wake up at 2 or 4 am and was unable to get back to sleep but the quality hours helped and I could tell in how I felt. This also reduced my frustration when I did wake up earlier than planned because I had been able to benefit from the golden hours.

- For shift workers, how can you maximize these hours of high-quality sleep?

- Can you arrange your day to make use of these optimal sleep times?
- Even if your workload is high, could you go to bed by ten pm and if you woke early and couldn't fall back to sleep, get up and dig into the work load with a more clear mind?

EIGHT

What to Avoid So You Can Fall Asleep

Being ready for sleep may require some advanced planning. It also may require that you stop doing some activities too close you your bedtime. Ideally, you want to create a routine that your body knows well and when you begin your routine, your body begins to anticipate the opportunity to sleep.

- Make sure you create a space for sleeping. Refer to the morning and nighttime routines below and try to create a space where merely walking into the room lets your body know it is time to sleep.
- No caffeine six hours prior to when you are going to be trying to sleep. The half-life of caffeine is six-eight hours, so factor that into your planning and keep in mind that everyone has different caffeine sensitivities. Know yours and adjust accordingly. If you drink more coffee than you need just out of habit, consider

switching to a herbal tea so you aren't getting the caffeine.

- No fluids for ninety minutes before going to bed.
- If your head is swimming, write things down and do a brain dump so you can shut your mind down.
- Place your phone and devices in another room.
- Use night lights, not room lights, to guide yourself if you need to use the facilities at night. Keep things dark. Light causes a shift in your hormones that you want to avoid unless it is time to get up. (Also orange lights, are more relaxing.)
- Exercising too close to when you want to go to sleep may be too stimulating to welcome sleep when it is time. For some, it is not an issue, so find out what works for you but be aware that this could impact your ability to fall asleep. Exercise does improve the quality of your sleep as long as it is not done too close to bedtime.
- Alcohol may help you fall asleep (or pass out), but it doesn't do anything to support quality sleep. Ideally, if you drink alcohol you want it out of your system before you fall asleep and it takes roughly one hour to digest one drink, two hours for two drinks, and so on — alcohol metabolizing as you sleep disrupts your sleep.
- No B Complex supplements after 3 pm (and if you are a shift worker, take them at the start of your "day").

- Avoid playing video games, especially from midnight to dawn and mid-afternoon, which are your prime sleep times. You should be napping!
- If coming off a nightshift, avoid light. Sunglasses and blue light blocking glasses are essential. You don't want the sunlight to kick up the melatonin suppression. You want that melatonin to begin winding you down.

NINE

Create An Environment and Routine for Sleep Checklist

If your sleep is impaired, so is your life to some degree. So addressing your sleep needs first is essential to overall well being.

Morning Routine (Adjust for Shift Work)

- Upon waking, meditate for 5-10 minutes. Use apps like Insight Timer or Calm to find some you enjoy. Start small and understand that meditation doesn't mean you will not have bouncing thoughts. It can be frustrating for people who have never done it. Start small.
- Do 5-10 minutes of exercise. There are some great 7 minute apps for bodyweight workouts that you can do in your home.
- Have a healthy breakfast. If you start your day with high sugar, you start these spikes where you need more sugar, and then you crash and then you reach for more sugar. Avoid that!

- Get some direct sunlight. Fifteen minutes of sunshine in the morning – turns off the melatonin production, so you feel less sleepy and sets up your other hormones to begin doing their jobs.
- Considering grounding or earthing when you wake up. Many of my clients get their feet on the earth as they sip their first coffee, and they feel it has improved their start to their day. They energy we create in our lives first thing, sets the tone for the day so try to avoid "panic mode."

Evening Routine (Adjust for Shift Work)

- Set the alarm to BEGIN your sleep time routine. Stop thinking you can do one more thing.
- Have a bedtime routine that unwinds you. Also, work towards clearing out your room so that the only associations you have with your bedroom are sleep and sex. TV's give off light that decreases melatonin so TV should be watched another time in another room.
- Sleep in comfortable clothing.
- Cool down the room (62-68 degrees).
- Blackout curtains for your bedroom.
- Darken the bathroom and avoid turning lights on when you go to the bathroom. Nightlights are sufficient. Use an orange light, not white.

- Wear earplugs/install sound-absorbing curtains.
- Play white noise to block out distractions.
- Turn off the phone and the cell phone
- A small snack before bedtime so you are not going to sleep hungry, nor stuffed.
- Five minutes of self-massage to turn off the sympathetic nervous system and turn on the parasympathetic nervous system can also help.
- Stay off devices for at least 60-90 minutes before bedtime and away from blue light or use blue light blocking glasses if you must be on light devices.
- Read a book, meditate, journal, take a hot bath or shower, have a cup of decaf tea (chamomile), and listen to a relaxing playlist or podcast/audiobook. Avoid anything exciting or stressful.
- You can use journaling as a way to make sure you write down everything that is swimming around in your head that you are afraid you will forget by morning so you can shut off your brain without having your thoughts go around and around all night long.
- Also, make sure you have soft lighting in your "wind down spaces" to encourage your body to begin shutting down for sleep. Avoid blue lighting and lean towards use of low-blue bulbs, orange and red lighting (salt lamps, candles, dim lights).

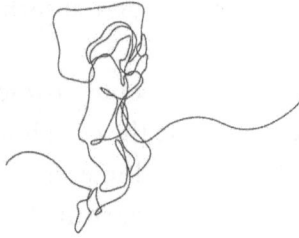

Additional Tips

- Schedule in your sleep first based on your schedule: remember that sleep prior to ten pm and early morning - as well as siesta times - is the most restorative sleep so take advantage of it if you can.
- It may take some time to be able to sleep and wake on your schedule so you can adjust it slowly each day until you are on plan. Develop a routine where possible and stick to it even on weekends or days off.
- Use of liquid Calcium and Magnesium in a 2:1 ratio 3 hours before bed.
- Have some plants in your room for increased air quality.
- Consider the creation of a sleeping room if you are trying to sleep when your household is awake and moving through their days.

You may not get it right the first few tries, just keep tweaking things and realize it may take a bit of time to correct some issues. Be reflective, you will know what is working for you, your schedule, your household, and your relationships. If you experience pressure from housemates, gently remind them that keeping a sleep schedule will make you a healthier and happier human and it will likely improve many facets of everyone's life!

TEN

Napping Tips

Naps can help reduce fatigue, and they are ideal when you have had less than eight hours sleep during your "nighttime sleep" or when it has been disrupted by periods of being awake or restless sleep. If you are at the point where you can sleep at any time and any place, you are likely critically fatigued.

We want to avoid the "mack truck" naps, where you wake up on the couch after 5 hours, sweating and stuck to the couch and trying to claw your way out of the thick brain fog, wondering what your name is and what yea rituals is.

NappaLatte

Take a cup of black drip coffee. Add three ice cubes and slug it – close your eyes for 20-25 minute power nap. This can provide a solid four hours of energy and focus. The caffeine will kick in, shift some other hormones, and wake you up.

Length of Naps

There are two types of naps that I want to address.

- 20-25 minute power nap or
- the 90 minutes, which is a full cycle of sleep. (Keep this in mind if you wake early from a regular night's sleep but can't do another 90 minutes before alarm sounds. Waking up mid cycle is hard!)

If you are napping to prepare for a work shift, planning to sleep more than 90 minutes but less than a second full cycle (and additional 90 minutes) will leave you fighting mental cobwebs and feeling worse because you are awakening out of an incomplete sleep cycle. That should pass after about fifteen minutes, and the benefits of the additional sleep will remain.

In the Latin culture, the siesta is typically mid-afternoon when there is a slight drop in core body temperature, which releases melatonin. If you have the chance to nap in the afternoon, it will be easier to fall asleep because of this. Plan accordingly.

Also napping for a sleep cycle before a night shift is beneficial. Avoid napping if your regular sleep time is coming and go to bed earlier so you can enjoy sustained sleep and back to back sleep cycles.

If you find yourself sleepy and can't nap, then go outside for a quick sunshine break if you can because that turns off the melatonin and begins a wake-up process.

Try one thing, pay attention to how you feel and tweak as needed before implementing the next suggestion.

ELEVEN

Conclusion

It is essential that you prioritize your sleep so that you can fall asleep, stay asleep, and enjoy good quality, restorative sleep. Sleep deprivation is a chronic issue in our society partially because we have glamourized this workaholic way of life and compress more work into our days while cutting into sleep time.

This short read is a quick overview of many things that you need to consider when cleaning up your sleep habits. If you are a shift worker, I highly recommend reading *21 Tips For Beating Fatigue And Improving Your Health, Happiness And Safety* by Dr. James Miller because he deals specifically with the issues that arise from various shift work systems.

Above all, do what you can and try all the suggestions *even* if you do not think they will work. Morning and evening sleep routines have been instrumental in getting me back to sleep and well-rested. But what works for one person, may not worth for another so be prepared to try different things.

If we don't change our environments then the changes will likely not stick. Make sure that the routines you want to establish are supported by environmental changes as well. If you are looking at your life holistically, you will be examining it from many perspectives and that will make the greatest impact on your success.

Sweet dreams.

TWELVE

Resources

Huffington, Arianna. *The Sleep Revolution: Transforming Your Life, One Night at a Time.*

Miller, Dr. James C. 2013. *21 Tips For Beating Fatigue And Improving Your Health, Happiness And Safety.*

Stevenson, Shawn. 2016. *Sleep Smarter: 21 Essential Strategies to Sleep Your Way to A Better Body, Better Health, and Bigger Success.*

Kathy Smart: *Sleep the Final Frontier Presentation.* CanFitPro. www.livethesmartway.com

About the Author

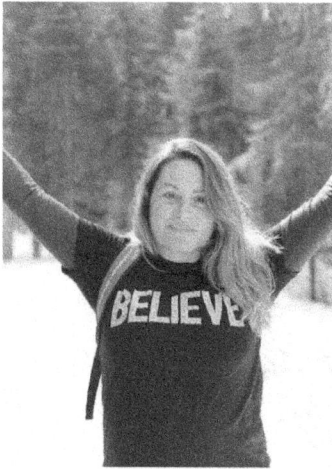

Jennifer is an author, speaker, life strategist and reiki master. When her own life hit the skids and she had to develop a new set of skills and tools to navigate unchartered waters, she realized how critical these skills where to her well-being.

Jennifer has spent over a decade studying how people think, talk, and act and how this impacts the quality of their lives and happiness. She can be found online at www.jennifersparks.ca.

Jennifer is also the author of several other books including *WTF to OMG: The Frazzled Female's Guide to Creating a Life You Love, Happy on Purpose, The Gratitude Transformation Journal,* and the soon to be released *50 Shades of Happy: How to Master Your Thinking and Dominate Your Day.* She is also the creator of the *LIFEMAP Infinity Planner* and the *LIFEMAP Quest Program.*

www.ingramcontent.com/pod-product-compliance
Lightning Source LLC
Chambersburg PA
CBHW021339290326
41933CB00038B/986